BEI GRIN MACHT SICH IHR WISSEN BEZAHLT

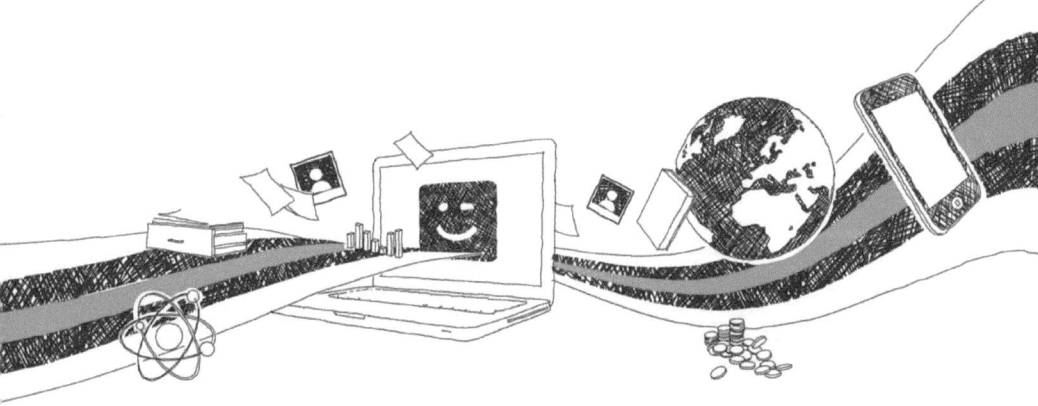

- Wir veröffentlichen Ihre Hausarbeit,
  Bachelor- und Masterarbeit

- Ihr eigenes eBook und Buch -
  weltweit in allen wichtigen Shops

- Verdienen Sie an jedem Verkauf

Jetzt bei www.GRIN.com hochladen und kostenlos publizieren

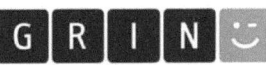

Marine Stephen Kimaro

Cerebral Palsy in children of Ohangwena region (Namibia): A case control study of risk factors

GRIN Verlag

Bibliografische Information der Deutschen Nationalbibliothek:

Die Deutsche Bibliothek verzeichnet diese Publikation in der Deutschen National-
bibliografie; detaillierte bibliografische Daten sind im Internet über http://dnb.d-
nb.de/ abrufbar.

Impressum:

Copyright © 2011 GRIN Verlag, Open Publishing GmbH
Druck und Bindung: Books on Demand GmbH, Norderstedt Germany
ISBN: 978-3-640-95835-1

Dieses Buch bei GRIN:

http://www.grin.com/de/e-book/168144/cerebral-palsy-in-children-of-ohangwena-
region-namibia-a-case-control

GRIN - Your knowledge has value

Der GRIN Verlag publiziert seit 1998 wissenschaftliche Arbeiten von Studenten, Hochschullehrern und anderen Akademikern als eBook und gedrucktes Buch. Die Verlagswebsite www.grin.com ist die ideale Plattform zur Veröffentlichung von Hausarbeiten, Abschlussarbeiten, wissenschaftlichen Aufsätzen, Dissertationen und Fachbüchern.

Besuchen Sie uns im Internet:

http://www.grin.com/

http://www.facebook.com/grincom

http://www.twitter.com/grin_com

MARINE KIMARO

CEREBRAL PALSY IN CHILDREN OF OHANGWENA REGION (NAMIBIA)

A CASE CONTROL STUDY OF RISK FACTORS

A FINAL RESEARCH PROJECT

TO THE ACADEMIC DEPARTMENT OF

THE SCHOOL OF SCIENCE AND ENGINEERING

IN PARTIAL FULFILLMENT OF THE REQUIREMENTS FOR THE

DOCTOR OF PHILOSOPHY DEGREE (PhD)

IN

PHYSICAL THERAPY

ATLANTIC INTERNATIONAL UNIVERSITY

HONOLULU, HAWAII (USA)

2011 – 2012

STRUCTURE OF THE PROJECT

PRELIMINARY PART

Title page

Acknowledgements

Contents

Abstract

BODY OF THE THESIS

List of Figures

List of Tables

Chapter I INTRODUCTION

Chapter II THESIS STATEMENT

Chapter III APPROACH/METHODS

- III.1 Research methodology

- III.2 Study area and study population

- III.3 Data collection and sources of data

- III.4 Ethical considerations

Chapter IV RESEARCH FINDINGS AND DISCUSSION

CONCLUSION PART

Chapter V CONCLUSIONS AND RECOMMENDATIONS

References

Bibliography

Mini – Curriculum Vitae (CV) with list of publications

Acknowledgements

My sincere thanks to the Academic Department of Atlantic International University (AIU) and my Academic Advisor Dr. Lucia Gorea for her immense academic assistance during the introductory coursework, research and thesis stages. Without her support I would not have achieved this success. My thanks too go to Ms.Nadia Bailey as my student counselor.

Acknowledgements to the Ministry of Health and Social Services - Ohangwena Health Directorate (Namibia) for allowing me to use their health facilities for interviews and research, thanks to Ohangwena Health Director Ms. Kaino Pohamba for technical support, lastly I sincere appreciate the cooperation I received from Cerebral Palsied children of Ohangwena region together with their parents and/or guardians, medical rehabilitation workers of Ohangwena region, my family. If I have forgotten to thank someone this is not intentional.

Contents:

List of Figures

List of Tables

Chapter I Introduction

Chapter II Thesis Statement

Chapter III Approach/Methods

- III.1 Research methodology

- III.2 Study area and study population

- III.3 Data collection and sources of data

- III.4 Ethical considerations

Chapter IV Research findings and Discussion

Chapter V Conclusions and recommendations

References

Bibliography

Mini - Curriculum Vitae with list of publications

Abstract:

In terms of neurological disorders, cerebral palsy is one of the most common conditions treated by medical rehabilitation professionals. In Ohangwena region (Namibia) the incidence of cerebral palsy (CP) is surpassed only by cerebral vascular accident (CVA). Cerebral palsy is a major cause of disability in children, affecting child's movement, posture and muscles tone.

Poor understanding of the etiology of CP, absence of steady decline in the percentage of cerebral palsied and dialogue whether home deliveries area major cause for CP necessitated a study to evaluate the risk factors associated with pathogenesis of cerebral palsy in young children.

A cross-sectional survey on the prevalence of cerebral palsy was conducted in young children aged one to five years in the three districts that formulate the region which is the area of the study. 62 cerebral palsied selected from medical rehabilitation departments patient register and 62 ages and sex matched neighborhood controls, all aged less than five (5) years were study subject matter. Qualitative design, using explorative and descriptive research strategies was the method of choice. Mothers were interviewed and at times additional information about the child was obtained from hospital patient records.

Findings were multi-faced; study revealed that antenatal (gestational) risk factors mainly associated with developed countries, were equally evident in Namibia a developing country, the case in point was maternal high blood pressure, and typical of developing world were factors like poor maternal nutrition (low protein intake during pregnancy) and low educational level of mother to mention the main ones.

In the case of whether home deliveries areas major cause of CP, the study found out incidence was at par between institutional and home deliveries. With regards to absence of steady decline in the percentage of CP, it was evident that modern improved obstetric and advanced perinatal care has resulted in the increased survival of low birth weight babies, which was not the case 20-30 years back.

Bottom-line Prevalence and clinical features of cerebral palsy in Ohangwena is comparable to other developing countries, as well as developed countries spreading in antenatal, perinatal and postnatal categories. Significant risk factors for cerebral palsy identified in the study are potentially modifiable.

Much study need to be done about CP as it is suggested anywhere from 20% - 50% of the real cause are not known. Support is needed to diagnosed children, family and the community in term of finance and social resources. As current there is no antenatal test for CP, no proven preventable measures in late pregnancy, and no known cure. To place more importance in gestational and perinatal care for mothers and babies will definitely reduce occurrence of cerebral palsy in young children population.

List of Figures:

Fig. 1: Quarterly recording of CP cases versus CVA

Fig. 2: Comparison of Home deliveries and Hospital deliveries

Fig. 3: Geographical position of Ohangwena Health Region

Fig. 4: Antenatal (Gestational) Risk Factors breakdown

List of Tables:

Chapter I INTRODUCTION

Cerebral Palsy (CP) is not a new disorder in terms of existence; there have probably been children with cerebral palsy since the beginning of human existence. Naturally a question will follow, if then is such an old disorder and not a disease, but a disability and it is known that in very rare and severe cases people die of overwhelming impact of physical impairment. Do these warrant clinicians, researchers and rehabilitation professionals to study cerebral palsy as a distinct medical condition?

The fact that cerebral palsy causes has been suggested to be anywhere from 20% to 50% unknown I believe more study is still needed. Evaluation of risk factors associated with cerebral palsy in children of Ohangwena Region (Namibia): case control study which is going be the main stay of my research and this thesis paper is an attempt to respond to the question posed in the just above paragraph of the introduction chapter.

Cerebral Palsy (CP) can be defined as a permanent disorder of movement and posture with sensory defects, due to brain damage or developmental abnormality occurring in fetal or early infancy. "Seven children are born with cerebral palsy per 100,000" (Bleck & Nagel, 1975:6)

Study done in Ohangwena Region (Namibia) has suggested that cerebral palsy etiology is poorly understood. Essentials indicators by Ministry Information System (MIS) and Statistics from Regional Medical Rehabilitation Departments indicates Cerebral Palsy as one of the most common neurological conditions treated by medical rehabilitation professionals in the region, surpassed only by Cerebral Vascular Accident (CVA) condition, this alone was a matter of concern that warranted a study to be conducted.

Another purpose of the study is to identify where explanation for the problem lies; whether it is within the health facilities deliveries or is the result of home deliveries facilitated by Traditional Birth Attendants (TBA's)? The chronic shortage of health professionals' doctors and nurses especially in the in rural (remote) health facilities does it contribute to the problem? And how this can be compared to the suggestions that perinatal and postnatal factors contributes majorly to cerebral palsy cases in developing countries, whereas in the developed (industrialized) countries cerebral palsy is mainly associated with ante-natal factors.

Though there are many associated markers or conditions associated with cerebral palsy, evidence of those conditions or risk factors don't guarantee that they are, indeed, the cause. In the 1970s obstetricians suggested that 'optimal' care (which they defined as emergency caesarean section for abnormalities on the electronic fetal monitor) then cerebral palsy would be avoided (Quilligan and Paul 1975). The outcome of their suggestion has had no effect on the rates of cerebral palsy (Stanley and Watson 1993, Nelson et al. 1996). Quilligan and Paul suggestion only increased caesarean rates and reduced rate of neonatal seizures. The point I am bringing home here is; that the question of the causes of cerebral palsy can as well be very tricky. Caesarean section may not be 'optimal' response. (Stanley, Blair & Alberman, p. 107)

With regards to not been a steady decline in the percentage of cerebral palsied children in the region, there is one important factor that has not clearly come to our recognition; the strides in the ability to keep alive and bring to health extremely premature infants has also increased the number of children who contract if you may allow cerebral palsy, whom 20 – 30 years back would have made it to their first birthday.

To assess, some of the identified risk factors for cerebral palsy, 62 cerebral palsied children were selected from medical rehabilitation department register; all aged less than five (5) years of age, residing in the region of Ohangwena were subject of study, against 62 age peer and sex matched from neighborhood as controls. *(Please note; it would have been ideal to have 250-300 children for the study to be standard, but the fact that Namibia being second only to Mongolia as far as the issue of population density is concerned, it was not practical, currently the Population of Namibia is approximately 2 million and is sparsely allocated)**

Information regarding antenatal, perinatal and postnatal was collected through interviewing mothers, wherever available, from hospital records of the study subjects. The impact of cerebral palsy to parents and immediate families, and social-economic issues associated was also another area of the study interest.

Chapter II THESIS STATEMENT

The outcome of early study done in the region, has suggest that cerebral palsy etiology is poorly understood. We all well know that knowledge is power. Once you have educate a person you have definitely empower him or her. So findings from the study opened a door for education and training on how to handle cerebral palsied children at home. (Number workshops were conducted in the region for parents and guardians of cerebral palsied children, these gatherings served as support groups as well). Importance of early therapy or intervention was explained, and parents/guardians were informed that the outcome of therapeutic intervention will very much depend on how early therapy starts and how extensive the brain damage is. *Signs* and *Symptoms* of a baby with cerebral palsy could be: *1.) a baby that is abnormally still and quiet or overactive with an irritable cry. 2.) Failure to suck properly 3.) Developmental milestones which do not develop properly 4.) Asymmetry – preferred movement of one or more limbs, while the other limbs are rather "lazy" and neglected.* It was explained and discussed. Parents/guardians were also informed that when it comes to neurological conditions, among which cerebral palsy is inclusive; that is much more difficult to correct abnormal habits than it is to prevent them from occurring. And that suitable response can be stimulated in the baby or child long before he/she is aware of co-operating.

Second problem statements was why number of cerebral palsy cases has and remain constantly high ranking among the Top 5 most conditions attended by medical rehabilitation professionals regional wise? Absence of steady decline in the percentage of cerebral palsied in the region needed a through explanation:

Statistics for the Period 2007 – 2009: <u>CVA versus CP (Top 2 diagnoses of Top 5)</u>

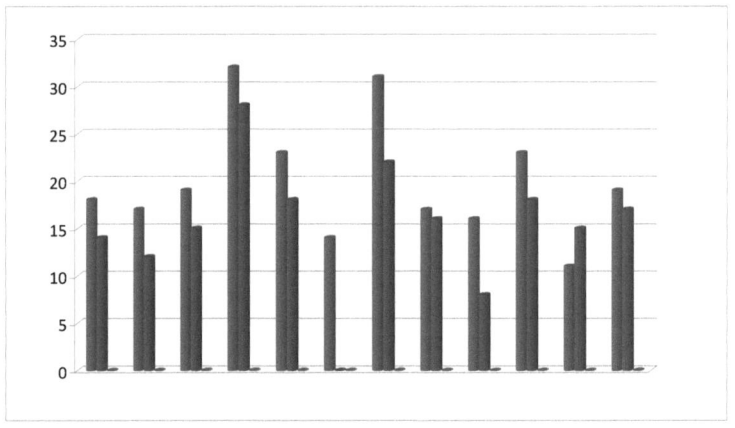

Fig. 1 [Blue column – CVA, Maroon column – CP]*

Note: Quarter 2 of the year 2008 – No CP case were recorded.

Quarter 3 of the year 2009 – CP case surpassed CVA cases.

The worries of the region not seen a steady decline in the percentage of cerebral palsied children is genuine. But, deep looks to the three (3) main district hospitals comparatively, reflects maternity wards that are relatively well equipped with trained human recourse. This explains the ability to keep alive and bring to health extremely premature infants, children born with Low birth weight (<1500g), the health section in the region has also witness children of gestational age <32 weeks, twin pregnancy and respiratory distressed surviving at a high rate. Whereas 20 – 30 years back when some these hospitals were not even there, and the ones which were there were not well equipped or having highly trained health staff. These shortfalls predispose number of children to cerebral palsy, whatever the case these children thanks to modern medical know-how they reach their first birthday and well beyond.

There is increasing evidence that cerebral palsy (CP) in developed countries results mainly from antenatal factors, whereas reports from developing countries suggest that perinatal and postnatal factors may be more important because of less than optimal delivery conditions. *(S. Al-Rajeh, O. Bademosi, A.Awada, H.Ismail, S. Al-Shammasi, A.Dawodu, DOI 10, 1111/j. 1469-8749 .tb14826.x, Nov 2008).* A study of 62 Ohangwena children with CP and comparison of their antecedent factors with those of a control group of 62 peers, the major risk factors identified were:

Gestational (Pregnancy) Risk Factors:

- Maternal high blood pressure
- Poor maternal nutrition (low protein intake during pregnancy)
- Incompetent cervix (premature dilation) leading to premature delivery
- Lower education level of mother
- Maternal "cold" with fever in their gestation
- History of CP in a sibling

Delivery Risk Factors:

- Delivery at home
- Illness during the first month of life
- Premature delivery (less than 37 weeks gestation)
- Prolonged rupture of the amniotic membranes for more than 24 hours leading to fetal infection
- Abnormal presentation such as breech, face, or transverse lie, which makes for a difficult delivery
- Severely depressed (slow) fetal heart rate during labour, indicating fetal distress
- Low APGAR score in five (5) minutes

Neonatal Risk Factors:

- Premature birth – the earlier in gestation the more likely he/she will be in risk of getting brain damage

- Asphyxia – insufficient oxygen to the brain due to breathing problems or poor blood flow in the brain

- Meningitis – infection over the surface of the brain
- Seizures caused by abnormal electrical activity of the brain

Thus, judging from Simple factor analysis and Multivariate analysis; Prevalence and clinical features of CP in Ohangwena region are comparable to those in the developed country. (Zhonghua Yu Fang *et al*, 2002 Sep; 36(5):323-6) Relevant risk factors could be seen primarily in gestational (antenatal), Delivery (perinatal) and Neonatal (post natal). In short risk factors might involve in mothers, children, environment and heredity. Bottom line what the study results suggests is: antenatal factors, perinatal and postnatal, play major role in the pathogenesis of CP in Namibia. Hence labeling developing countries as having "less than optimal delivery conditions" do not guarantee that they are, indeed the causes of cerebral palsy *per se*.

Table 1: Distribution of Cerebral Palsied Children per District, 2007 - 2009

NAME OF THE DISTRICT	NUMBER OF CP CHILDREN
EENHANA	19
ENGELA	23
OKONGO	20
TOTAL: (OHANGWENA REGION)	62

The question of Deliveries at Home was another area where Regional health authority was interested; exactly they wanted to know the role or rather the impact in the contribution to Cerebral Palsy.

Fig. 2: Home Deliveries and Hospital (Institutional) Deliveries

(SEE THE GRAPH BELOW)*

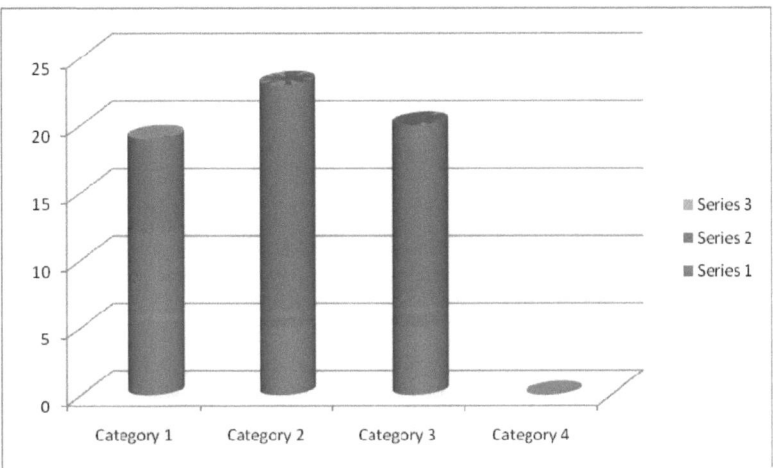

Category 1: Eenhana District (Blue=Home Delivery, Maroon=Hospital Delivery)*

Category 2: Engela District (Blue=Home Delivery, Maroon=Hospital Delivery)*

Category 3: Okongo District (Blue=Home Delivery, Maroon=Hospital Delivery)*

Simple factor analysis, cases of Cerebral Palsy incidence does not differ much between home deliveries and institutional deliveries.

Analysis done on general preference by Eenhana health district of home (birth) deliveries, by simple interview of the parents/guardian the main reason was distances from health facilities and financial constriction when it comes to hire a vehicle to ferry expecting mothers to hospital. Another reason that was not very common was the problem of teenagers who have been hiding pregnancy and as result opts for home deliveries.

The problem learned with home deliveries in the specific district in question and the rest of the districts that were subject of the study was; was a mix of unplanned home births and few planned home birth. The risk step in when was <u>unattended birth, high-risk homebirths</u> and <u>improper trained traditional birth attendants</u> with <u>limited equipments</u>.

Chapter III: APPROACH/METHODS

III.1 Research methodology

A qualitative design, using explorative and descriptive research strategies was used. Questions:

- Did the mother have "cold" with fever in their gestation?

- Educational level of the mother; which grade did you attains?

- Was the delivery home or institutional? If home why?

- Did your child got ill e.g. meningitis?

Other issues that appear to be more technical were read from hospital files of the child, whenever possible. The researcher then classified the responses provided to some of the identified risk factors for cerebral palsy.

III.2 Study area and study populations

The area of study was Ohangwena region, one of the thirteen health regions of the country. (Namibia):

Fig. 3: *Geographical position of Ohangwena Health Directorate*

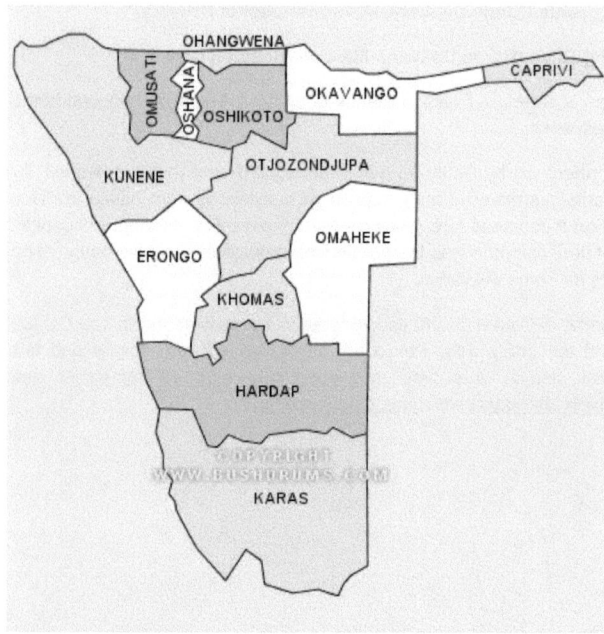

Three (3) participating districts namely Engela, Eenhana and Okongo composes Ohangwena region. Children with cerebral palsy born between the year 2005 and 2003, selected from medical rehabilitation departments registers of the regions three districts hospitals were the targeted population of the study. These were children who were < five (5) years of age, residents of Ohangwena region and cerebral palsy associated visual impairment, mental retardation, speech and hearing impairment, seizures and hyperkinesias. The control group was children who were cerebral palsy free, matched for sex and age, the first kid from neighborhood meeting these conditions was taken as control. All aged less than five (5) years and residing in Ohangwena region.

III.3 Data collection and sources of data

Data was collected through mother's interview regarding information about antenatal, perinatal and postnatal period. Wherever available, hospital records of the study subjects were scrutinized. Qualitative data was analyzed manually. The validity and/or reliability of the data were ensured by a pilot study done in Eenhana district. Resulting from pilot study some amendments were done to the research questions and data/information collection Form.

The Form designed for data collection was supplied to three (3) district hospitals medical rehabilitation departments, it had columns for:

- *Registration number:*
- *Name of the patient/client:*
- *Date of birth:*
- *Gender:*
- *Parent's/guardian name:*
- *Physical address:*
- *Type of labor (normal, assisted, other):*
- *Place of delivery (home or hospital):*
- *If the answer is home, was traditional birth attendant trained or not? :*
- *Pregnancy (First/Prima gravida? Or second etc.)? :*

III.4 Ethical considerations

Ethical perspective was also considered. Permission was obtained form the Regional Health Authorities to conduct a study within the ministry's facilities. Parents/guardians of study population and the control group were requested a permission before their participation in the study. The purpose of the research was thoroughly explained to them all. It was made clear to them that their participation in the study was voluntary, and they were free at any time to withdraw from the study at will.

Chapter IV: RESEARCH FINDINGS AND DISCUSSIONS

As it was reflected in the Thesis statement section, studies have suggested poor understanding of Cerebral Palsy etiology. Since the days of orthopedic surgeon William J. Little (1861) it was widely assumed that asphyxia due to poor obstetric care during labour and delivery has been implicated as a major cause of cerebral palsy. Ideas of "optimal obstetric care" interventions; aimed at reducing birth asphyxia and other birth complications have not resulted in lowering the rates of cerebral palsy. Of contrast, studies done recent have implicated antenatal and postnatal factors more than perinatal in the etiology of the cerebral palsy. Many factors, both genetic and acquired *(These include; hypoxic-ischemic injury, structural malformations, vascular disorders, intraventricular or subarachnoid hemorrhage, infections, hormonal disorders, toxins, trauma, metabolic disease, prematurity, hemolytic disease of the newborn)** have been postulated as causes of cerebral palsy. In recent years, a number of studies have sought to determine the relative contribution of these genetic and acquired factors to cerebral palsy. Modern improved obstetric and advanced perinatal care has resulted in the survival of large number of; *low birth weight* babies, children born with less than 1500gram [<1500] courtesy of medical advancement they reach their first birthday, this associated with an increased proportion of cerebral in these babies. *Children of gestation less than 32 weeks, twin pregnancy and respiratory distressed surviving at a high rate.* This could not be the case 20 – 30 years back. Namibia being one of the few developing countries where modern obstetrics and perinatal care are used to lesser extent compared to developed (industrialized) countries, in my opinion a cohort study would have been appropriate, but such studies are lengthy, and ask enormous resources, thus we opted for a case control study, geared at assessing some of the identified risk factors for cerebral palsy.

Another variable that study found to be *significantly associated with cerebral palsy was home delivery.* Eenhana health district during the study period *(January 2007 – December 2009)* had nineteen *(19) cases*, of which *twelve (12) cases were home deliveries. This means 63% of Eenhana's cases were home delivery. (i.e. 19% of the region's cerebral palsy caseload).* Since teenage pregnancy ranks high in Ohangwena region, maternal age at birth and birth order of the child were studied as possible contributors to cerebral palsy. The finding was: *Eight (8) out of 12 home deliveries were to mothers ranging from 13 – 17 years (teenagers).* Hence, confirms a statement that is in the thesis statement section that highlighted the issue of teenage pregnancies who later opted for home delivery after concealing their pregnancy. It should also been noted that birth order of these children was *prima gravida.* In the sister district of Okongo, quarter of 20 cases of noted cases were home delivery. (5 of 20 of the cases), 3 of the 5 were teenage pregnancy prima gravida, although statistically not significant, but assert the explanation of Eenhana health district.

Through the study conducted in Ohangwena region with regards to cerebral palsy risk factors – case control, *a school of thought that adhere to an increasing evidence that cerebral palsy CP) in developed (highly industrialized) results mainly from antenatal factors, while in the developing suggesting perinatal and postnatal factors courtesy of less than optimal delivery conditions.* The outcome of study suggests antenatal factors including; maternal high blood pressure, Lower level of education, Poor maternal nutrition (low protein intakes during pregnancy), and maternal "cold" with fever play a major role in the pathogenesis of cerebral palsy in Namibia.

Fig. 4: Antenatal *(Gestational) Risk Factors breakdown*

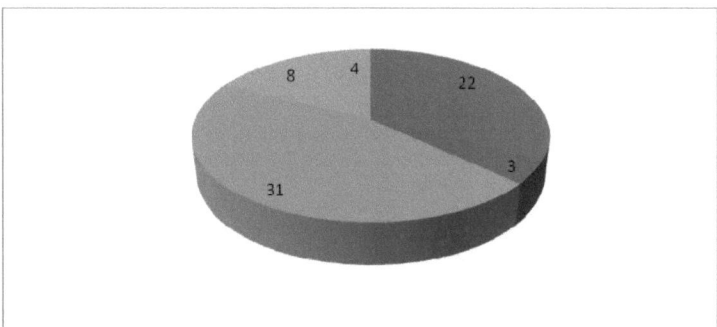

The above pie chart depicts risk factors during the antenatal period from the study that was conducted in Ohangwena region. 22 of 62 were categorized with **maternal high blood pressure.** 3 of 62 **poor maternal nutrition (low protein intakes during pregnancy). 31 of 62 were associated with lower level education, 8 of 62 suffered maternal "cold" with fever in their gestation.** While 4 of 62 had a **history of cerebral palsy in a sibling.** (This has also been the findings of S. Al-Rajeh *et al* 2008, and Quilligan and Paul 1975)

Chapter V: CONCLUSIONS AND RECOMMENDATIONS

Cerebral Palsy (CP) – is the most common neurological disorder in children. Study done for this paper, rates CP second only to Cerebral Vascular Accident (CVA) in the Ohangwena region. Epidemiological evidence suggests that antenatal origins area major cause. However, according a study conducted, suggests perinatal and postnatal factors playing substantial role equally as well. The study was able to suggest otherwise the concept that antenatal factors are the main cause of CP in developed countries, and perinatal and postnatal explains CP in developing countries. Study has found out that in the developing countries antenatal factors area substantial cause for cerebral palsy as well.

Study was able to establish, the explanation of steady rise in number of children with cerebral palsy. The notion that has been embraced long, of birth asphyxia as the main contributing cause to cerebral palsy, called for implementation of improved obstretic and advanced perinatal care. This in turn resulted in the increased survival of large number of low birth weight babies whom in the past would not have survive.

Significant risk factors for cerebral palsy identinfied in the study are potentially modifiable. The case of Low Birth Weight (LBW) could be prevented by nutrition, child spacing, educating expecting mothers to avoid doing heavy duty (overwork) during pregnancy.

Although this study place the incidence of cerebral palsy at par when comes to home delivery against institutional (hospital) delivery, taking into consideration lack of sufficient delivery instruments, high risk pregnancy and level of education and understanding of teenage pregnant mothers when deliver unattended, home delivery become risky and problematic at times especially in the rural area.

From the study done following are some suggested recommendations; the fact that CP causes has been suggested to anywhere form 20% - 50% unknown, and currently there is no antenatal test for cerebral palsy, no proven preventable measures in the late pregnancy and no cure, this situation remain wanting. More funds should be availed to support diagnosed child, and also their family and community. A cerebral palsied child require considerable social and financial support in their day lives.

Another recommendation is towards hospitals/clinics, although the records were available to a relative number of cases, the documentation was not to standard. A number of important parameters were lacking and at times the small that was available was not read-able. Proper documentation of events in antenatal, perinatal and postnatal period are very cardinal. An organized and standardized record keeping for all newly born, and if not practical at least for high risk babies.

I should be thankful to mothers who were interviewed, but I have a bit of reservation as a good number of mothers were not very free to give their antenatal history, fearing blames by their husbands, in-laws for the child's condition.

References (Bibliography):

1. Lindsay, B. Including Children with Cerebral Palsy. A & C Black Limited. London. 2008

2. Chang JJ, Wu Ti, Wu WL, Su FC. Kinematical measure for spastic reaching in children with cerebral palsy. Clin Biomech. 2005; 20:381-8

3. Miller, F. Physical Therapy of Cerebral Palsy. Springer and Science Business Media. USA. 2007

4. Bjorklund, R. Cerebral Palsy. Marshal Cavendish. London. 2007

5. Tebbet, K. Management of Cerebral Palsy – a transdisciplinary approach. SAGE Publications. USA. 2006

6. Miller, F., Bachrach, S.J. Cerebral Palsy – a complete guide to caregiving. The John Hopkins University Press. USA. 2006

7. Gordon, C., Charles, J., Steven, L., Wolf, PT., Methods of Constraint –induced therapy for children with hemiplegic cerebral palsy: development of a child-friendly intervention for improving upper-extremity function. Arch Phys Med rehabol. 2005; 86: 837-44

8. Ross, J., I Can't Walk but I can Crawl – living with Cerebral Palsy. Paul Chapman. USA. 2005

9. Workinger, M.S. Cerebral Palsy Resource Guide – for speech language pathologists. Thomson Delmar Learning. USA. 2005

10. Grimm, J., The Heart's Alphabet – daring to live with Cerebral Palsy. Tasora Books. USA. 2007

11. Odding, E., Roebroeck, M.E., Stam, H.J., The Epidemiology of Cerebral palsy: incidence, impairments and risk factors. Disabil Rehabil. February 28 2006; 28(4): 183-91 [Medline]

12. Lie, K.K., Gronholt, EK., Eskild, A. Association of Cerebral with Apgar score low and normal birthweights infants: population based cohort study. BMJ. 2010; 341: c4490 [Medline]

13. Moster, D., Wilcox, A.J., Vollset, S.E., Markestad, T., Lie, R.T. Cerebral Palsy among term and posterm births. JAMA. September 1 2010; 304(9): 976-82 [Medline]

14. Low, A.S., Lee, S.L. et al. Difficult with prenatal diagnosis of the Walker-Warburg Syndrome, Acta Radiol 46-645-65

15. Woodwar, L.J., Anderson, PJ., Austin NC, et al. Neonatal MRI to predict neurodevelopmental outcomes in preterm infants. N Engl J Med, Aug 17 2006; 355 (7): 685-94 [Medline]

Mini – Curriculum Vitae (CV) and list of publications:

Mr. Marine Kimaro

Mr. Kimaro has been a doctoral degree student at Atlantic International University (AIU), Honolulu, Hawaii (USA) since 2010. He received his Master's Degree (MA) majoring in Physiotherapy in 1988 from the Higher Insitute of Physical Culture *"G.Dimitrov"* (Now National Sports Academy *"Vassil Levski"*) in Sofia, Bulgaria. He has served as a senior and principal physiotherapist in the Ministry of Health and Social Services (Namibia) in different capacities as clinician, tutor and consultant since 1993. Currently is employed by the Directorate of Health – Ohangwena in Namibia, within the Health Ministry as a Regional Physical Therapist, heading a health program: "Disability Prevention and Medical Rehabilitation" (DPRS).

Publications:

e-book: **Pharmacotherapeutics**

Institution/College: Atlantic International University

Author: Marine Kimaro

Archive No.: VI56513

ISBN (E-book): 978-3-640-71933-4

DOI: 10.3239/9783640719334

Category: Essay

Language: English

Year: 2010

Website: http://www.grin.com/e-book/156513/pharmacotherapeutics